"WHAT'S WRONG WITH YOU?"

NICOLE YATES

Copyright © 2022 by Nicole Yates

All rights reserved.

No portion of this book may be reproduced in any form without written permission from the publisher or author, except as permitted by U.S. Copyright law.

Book Cover, Design, and Formatting by E. Rose Books. Madison, Wisconsin.

ISBN: 9798361514908

1st Edition 2022

Dedication

To Beefcake – who loved me before I knew who I was.

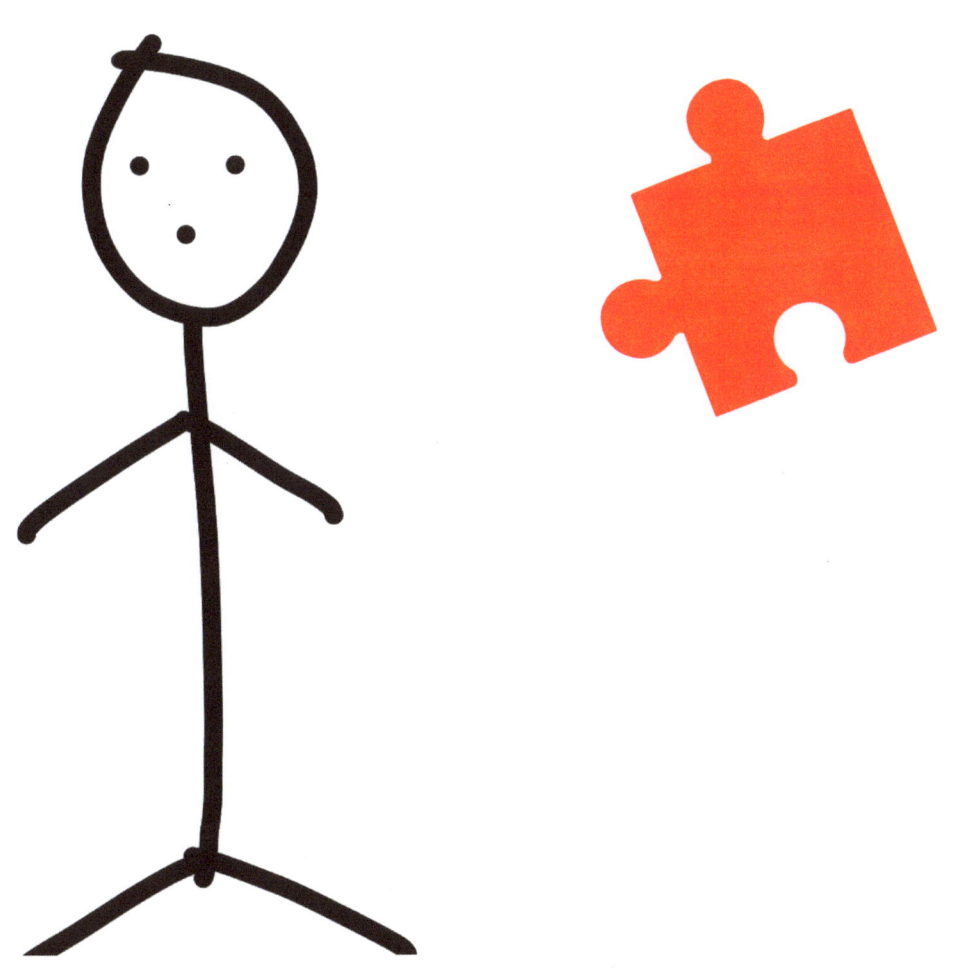

"What's wrong with you?"

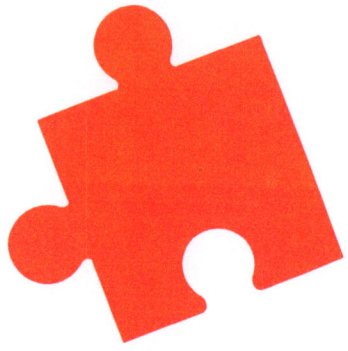

"You're not trying hard enough."

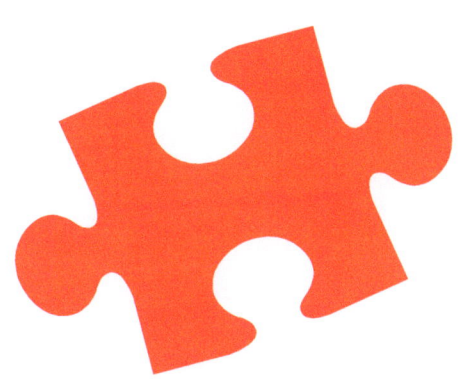
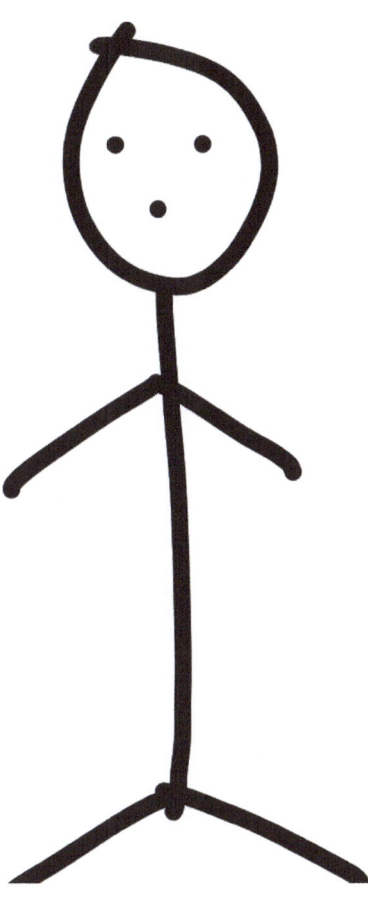

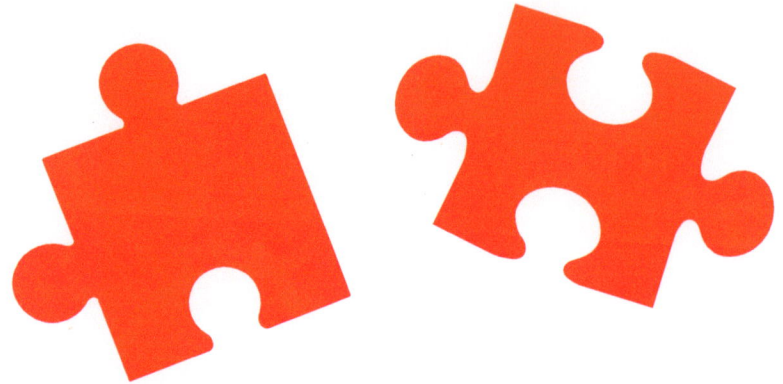

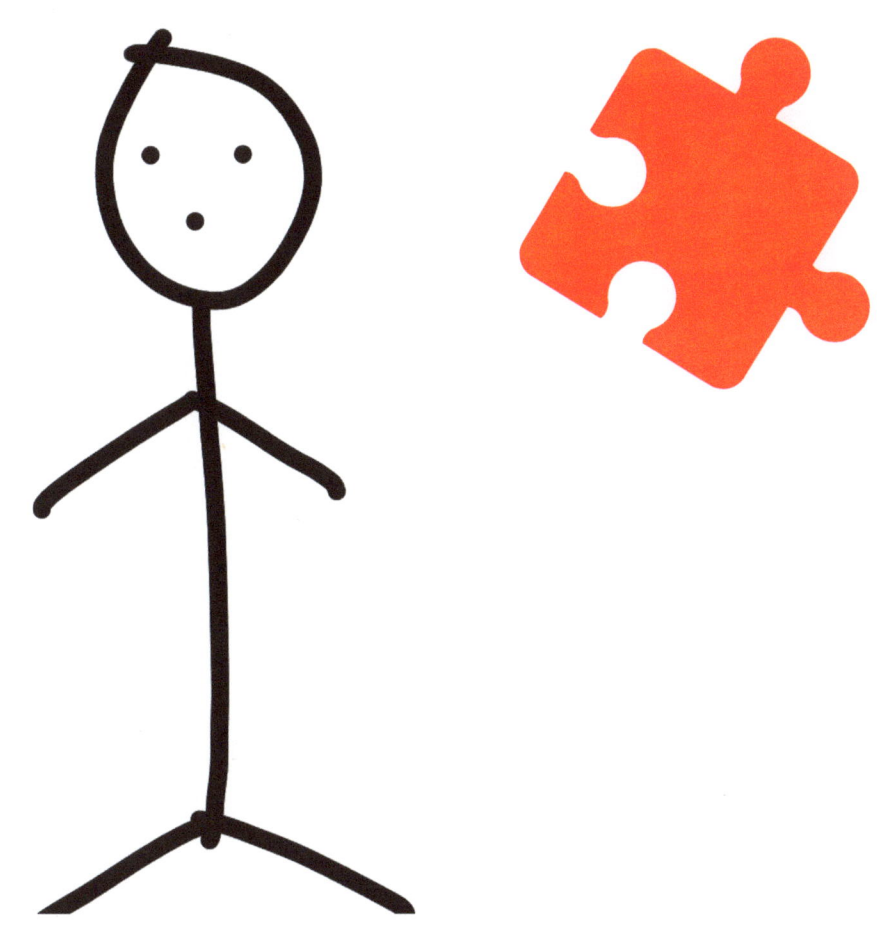

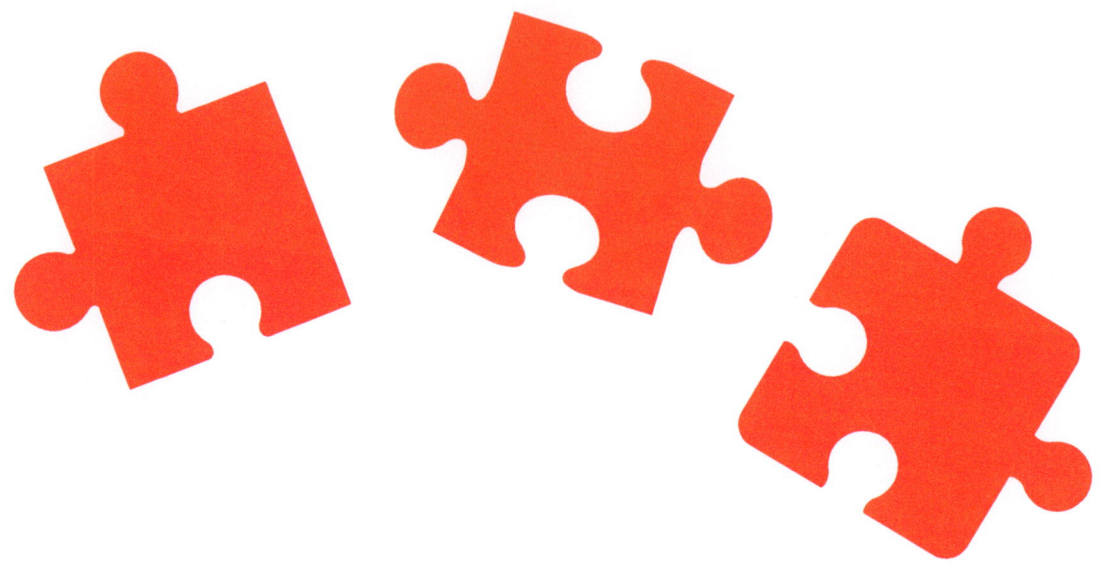

"Stop daydreaming."

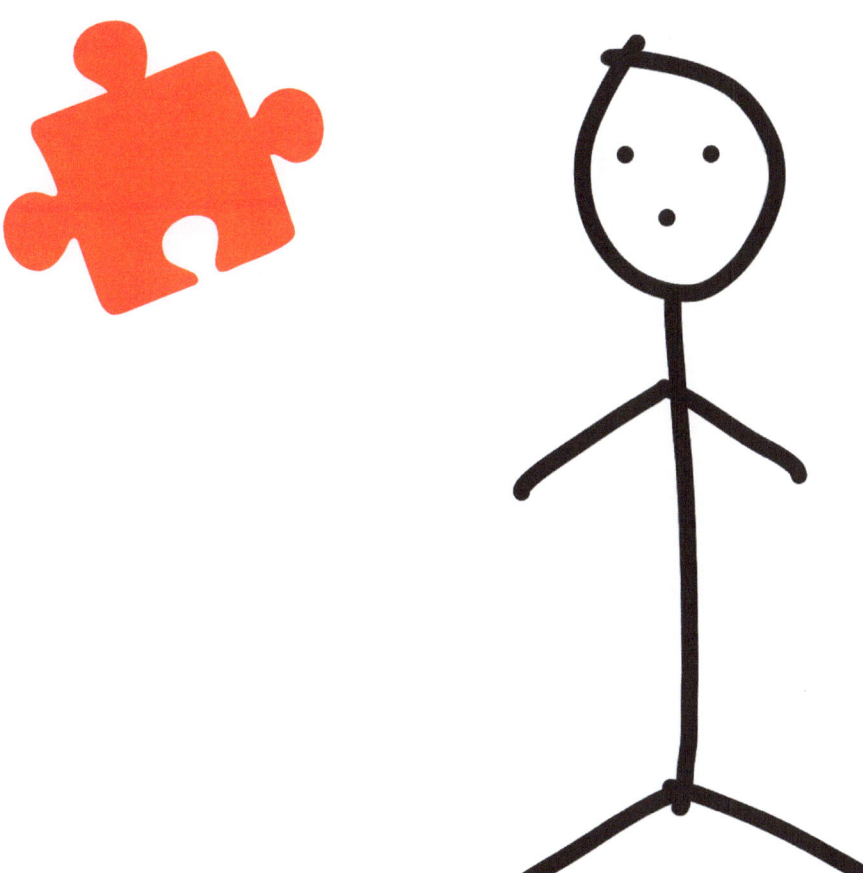

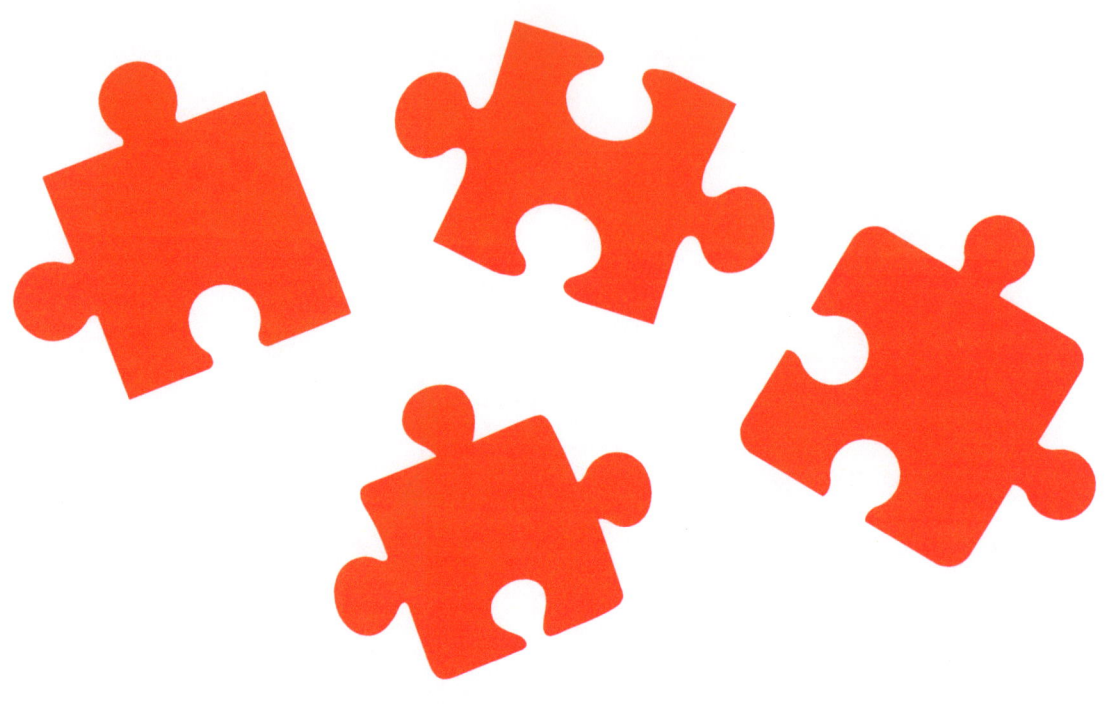

"You're better than this."

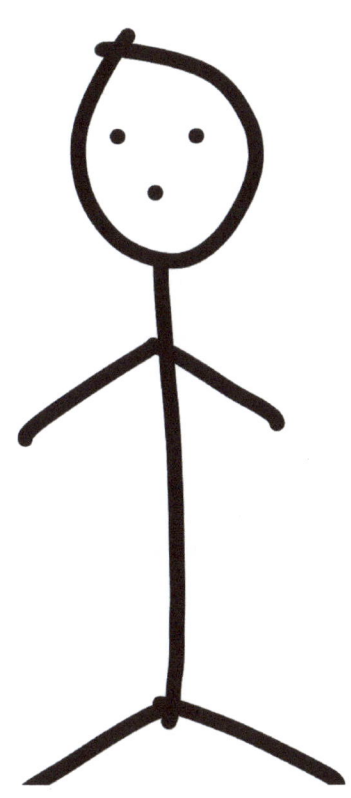
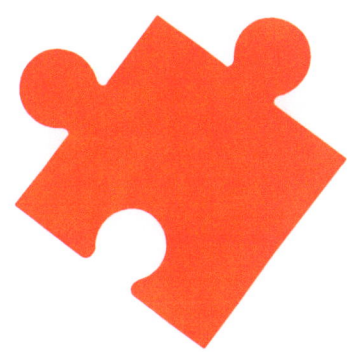

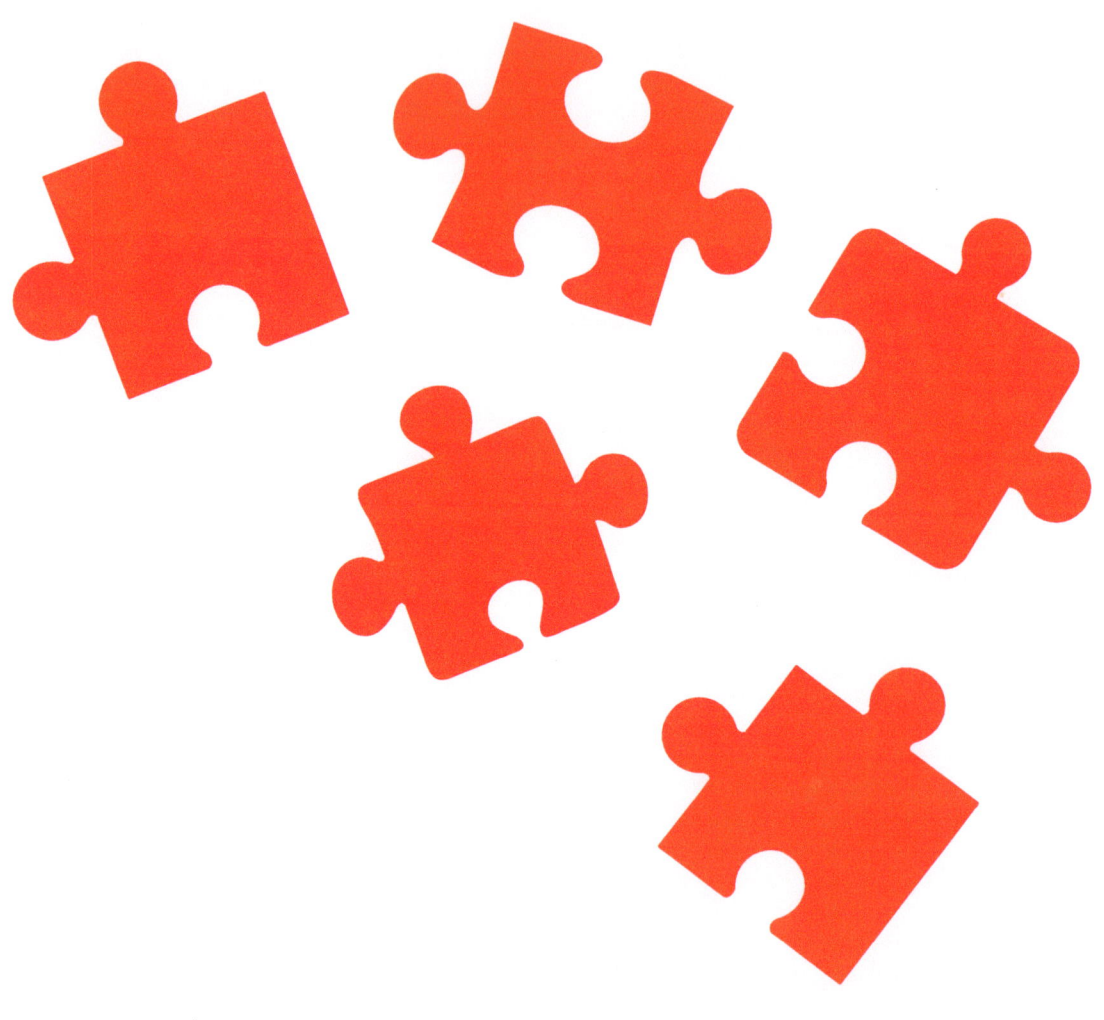

"Don't make a scene."

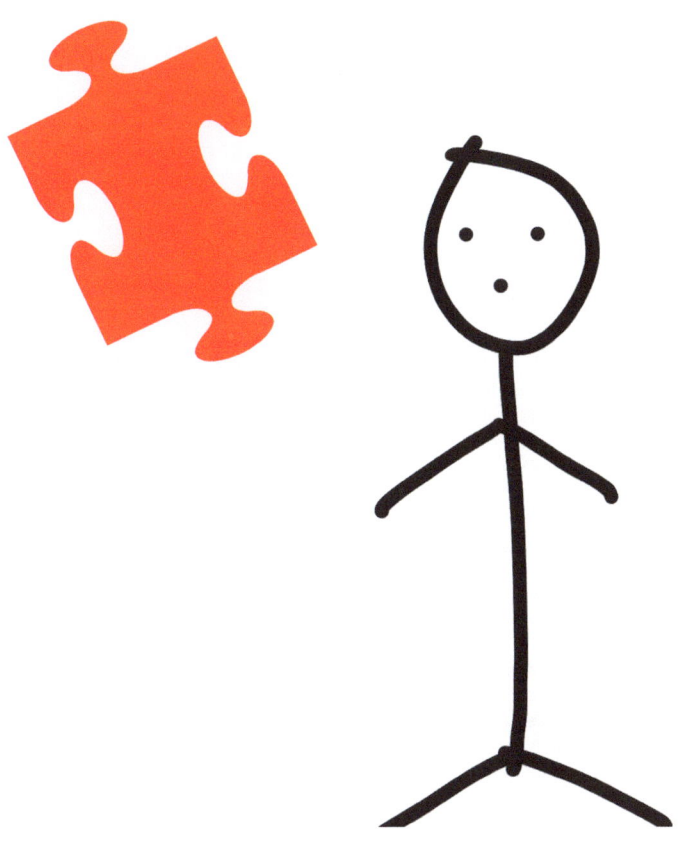

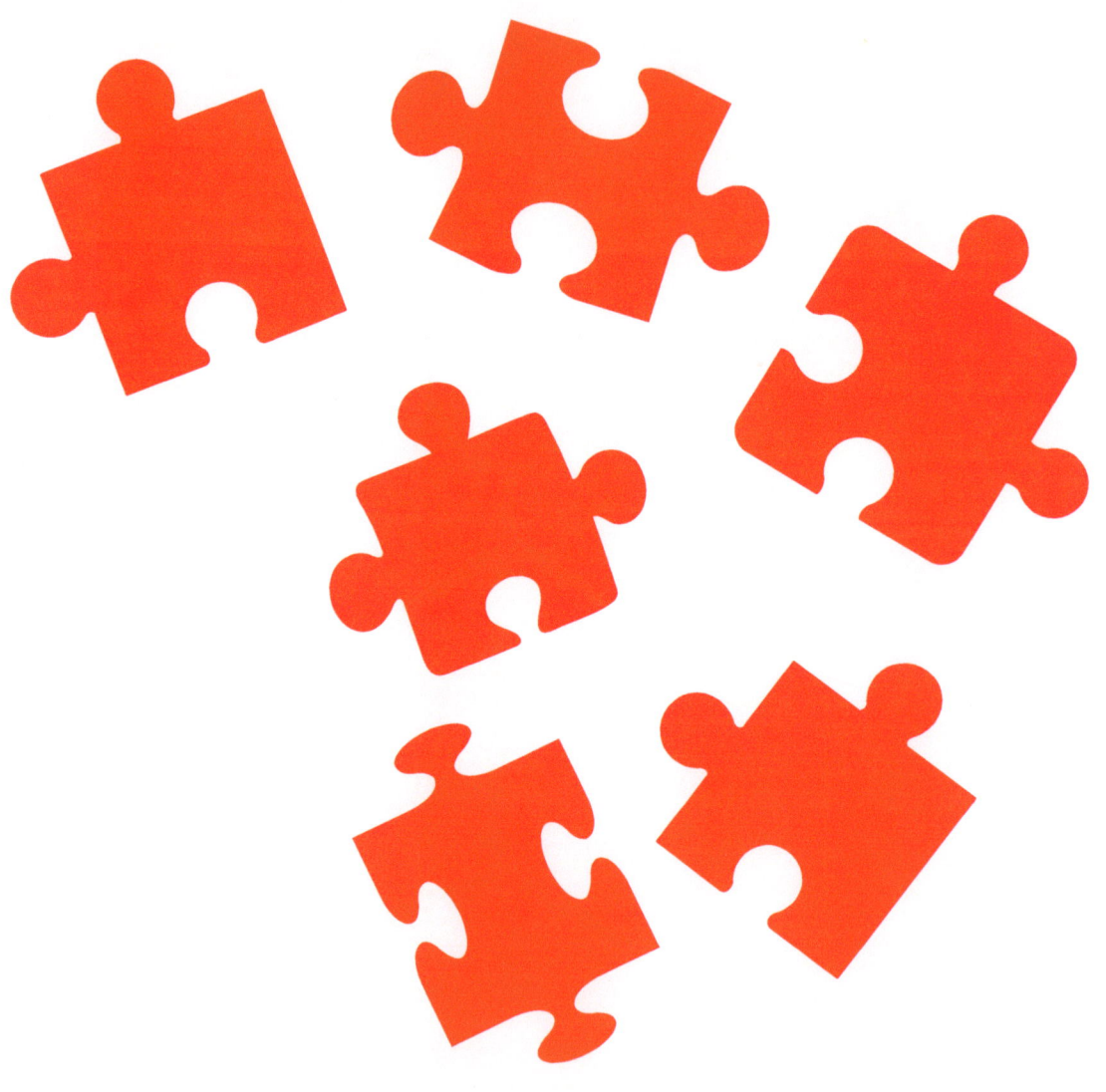

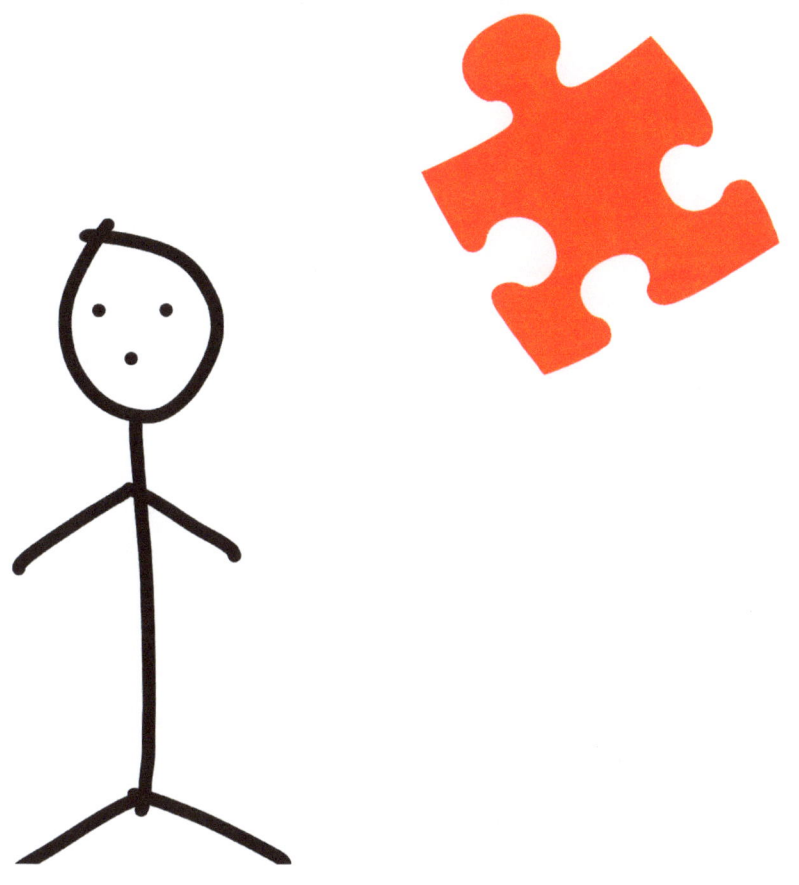

"You're not invited."

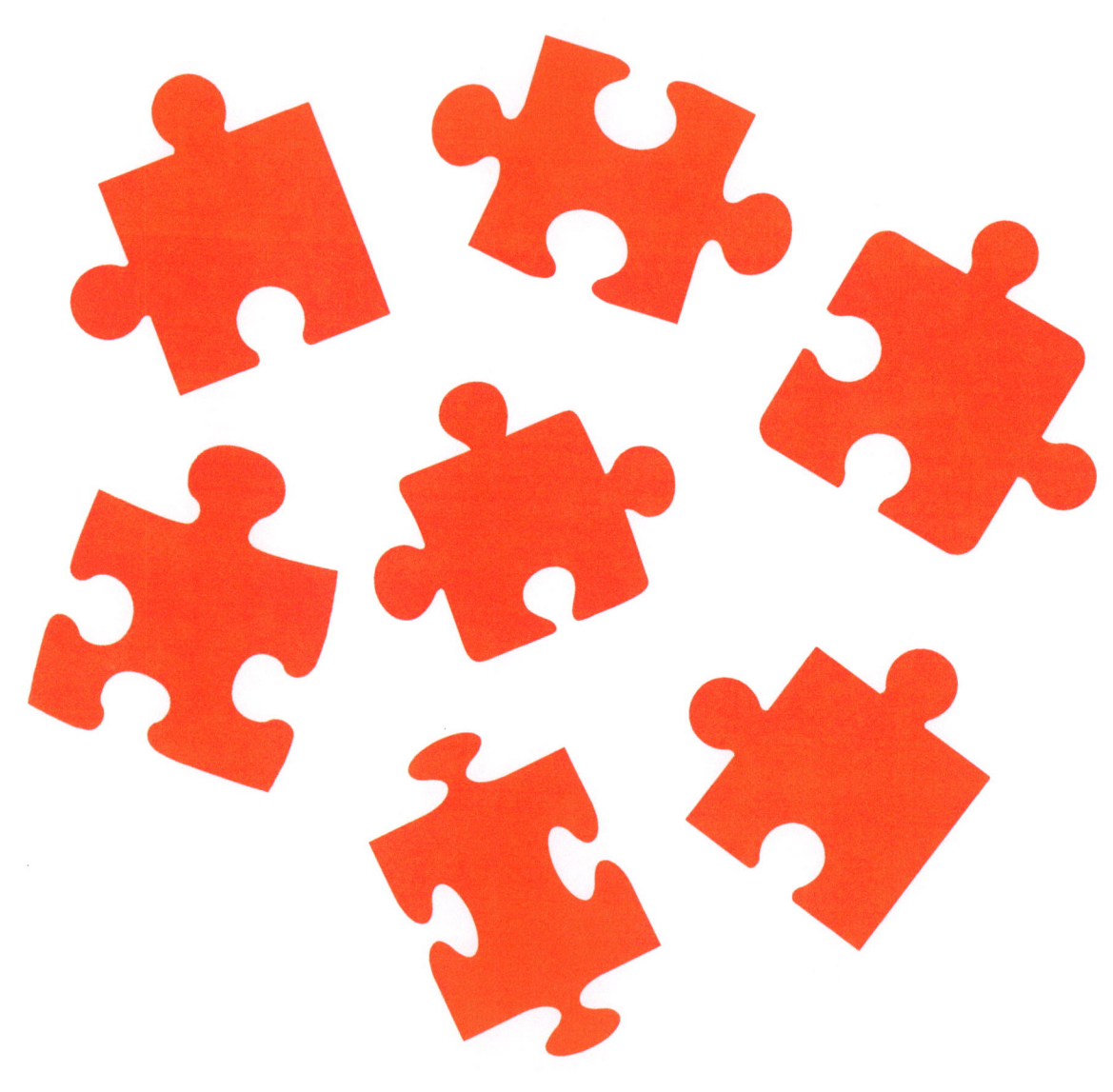

"It's all in your head."

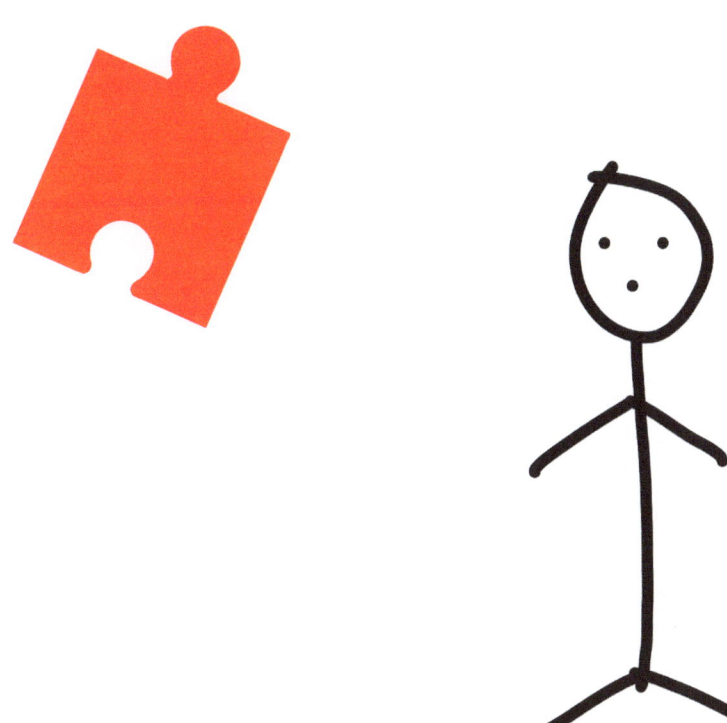

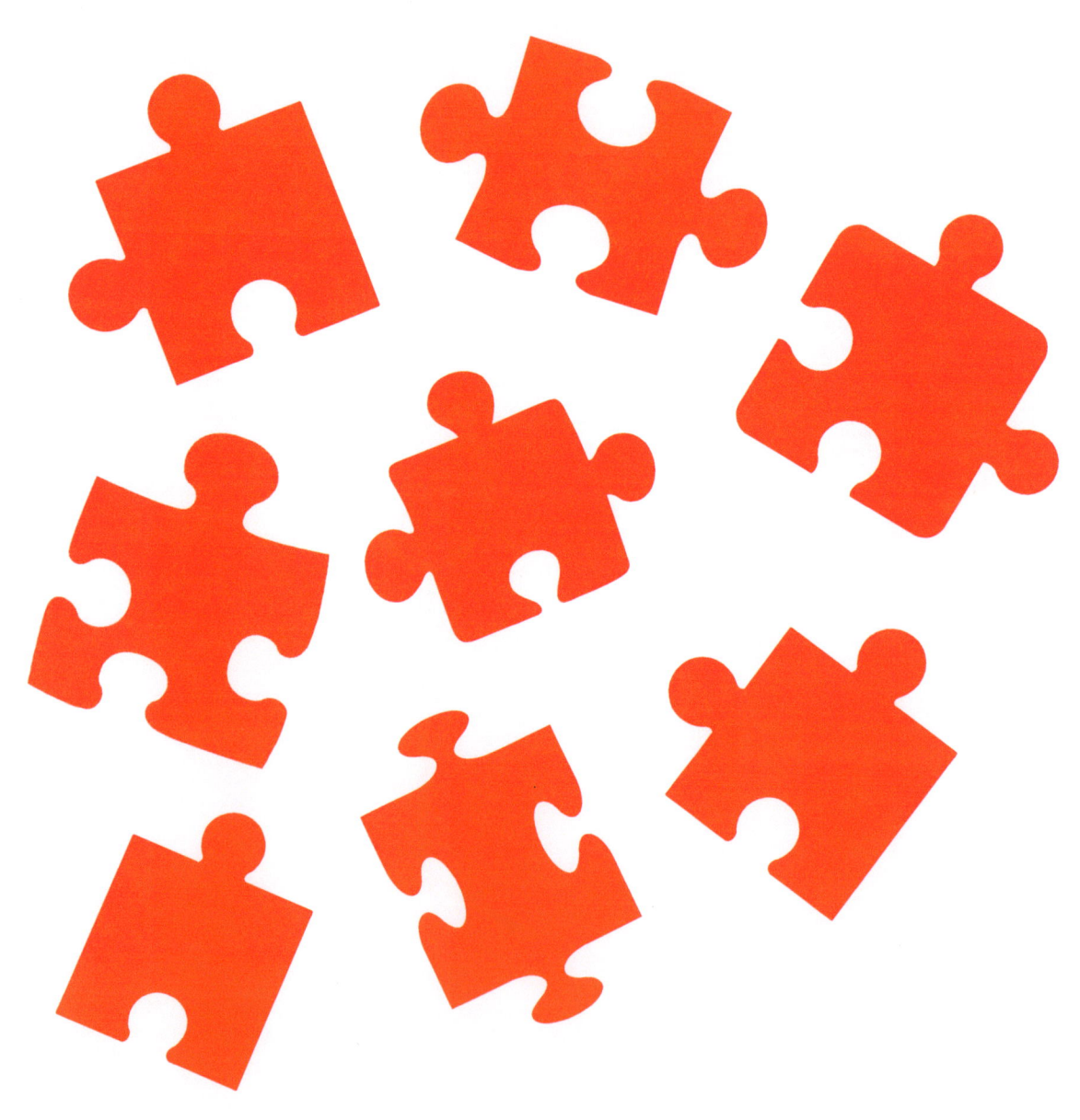

"Stop lying."

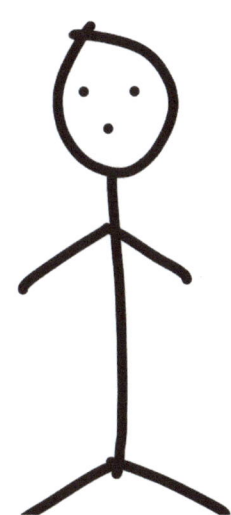

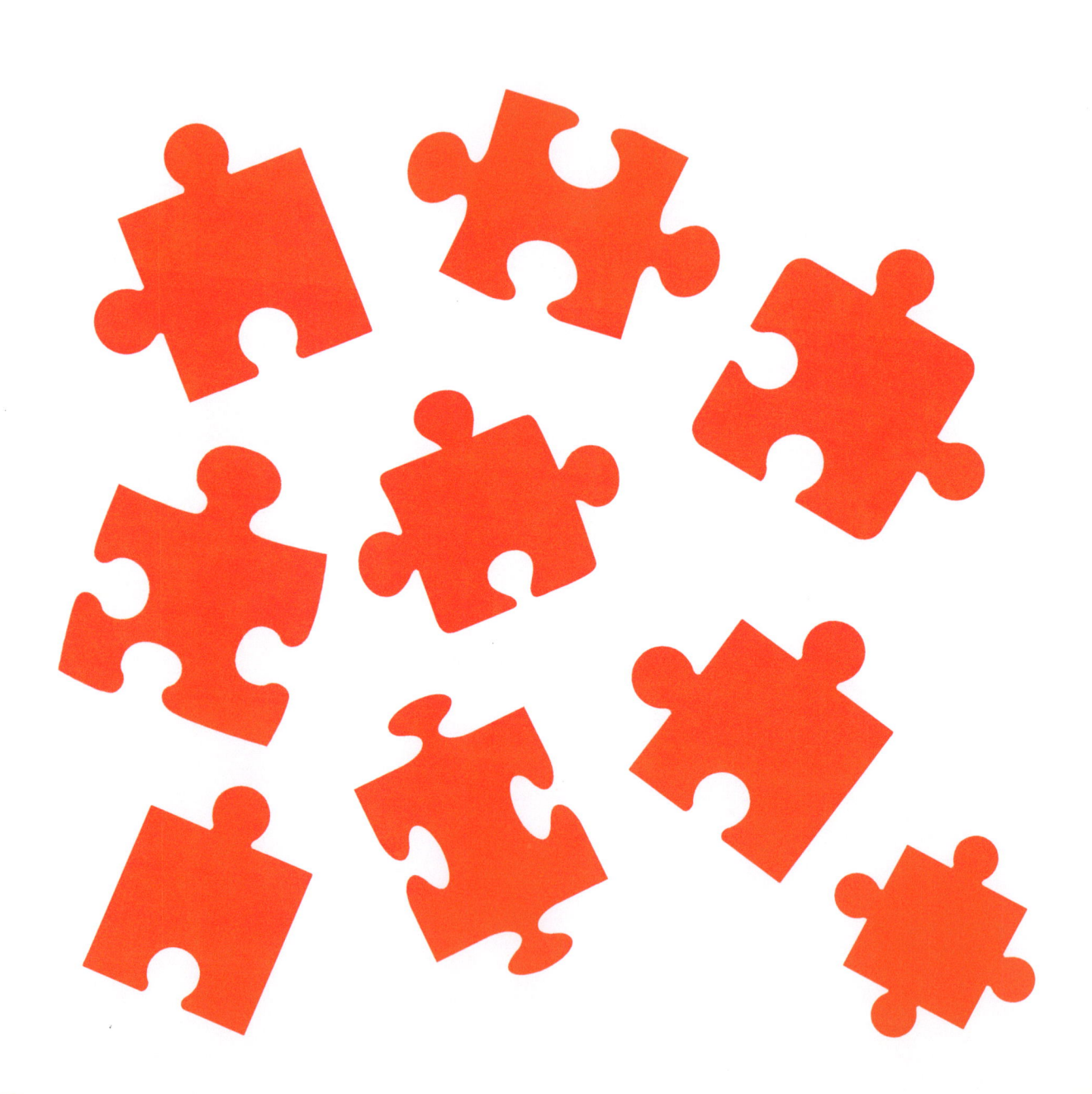

"I don't want to be with you."

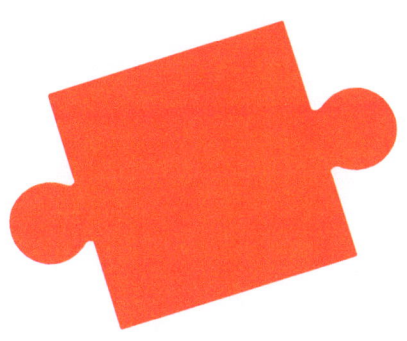
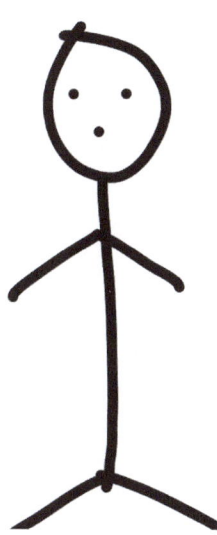

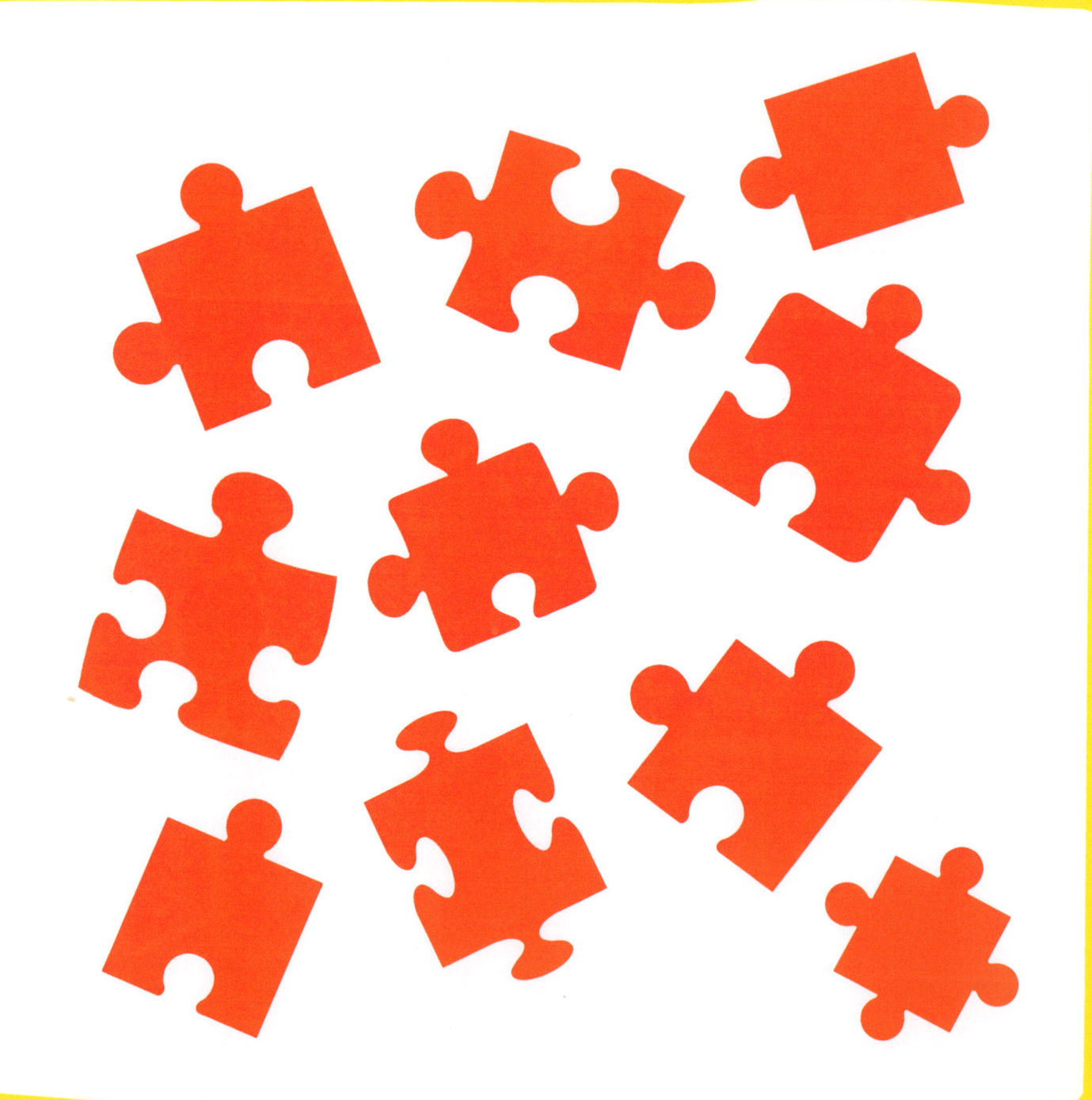

"You're fired."

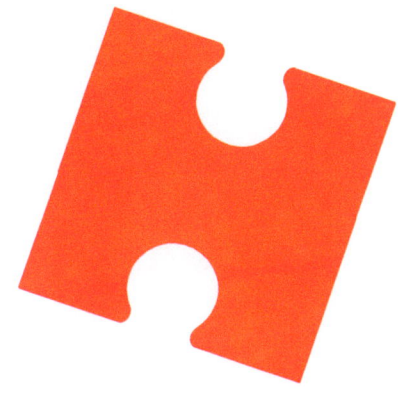
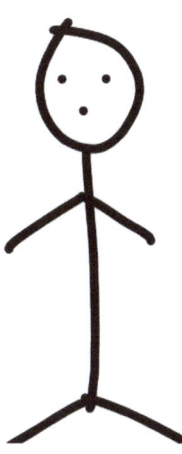

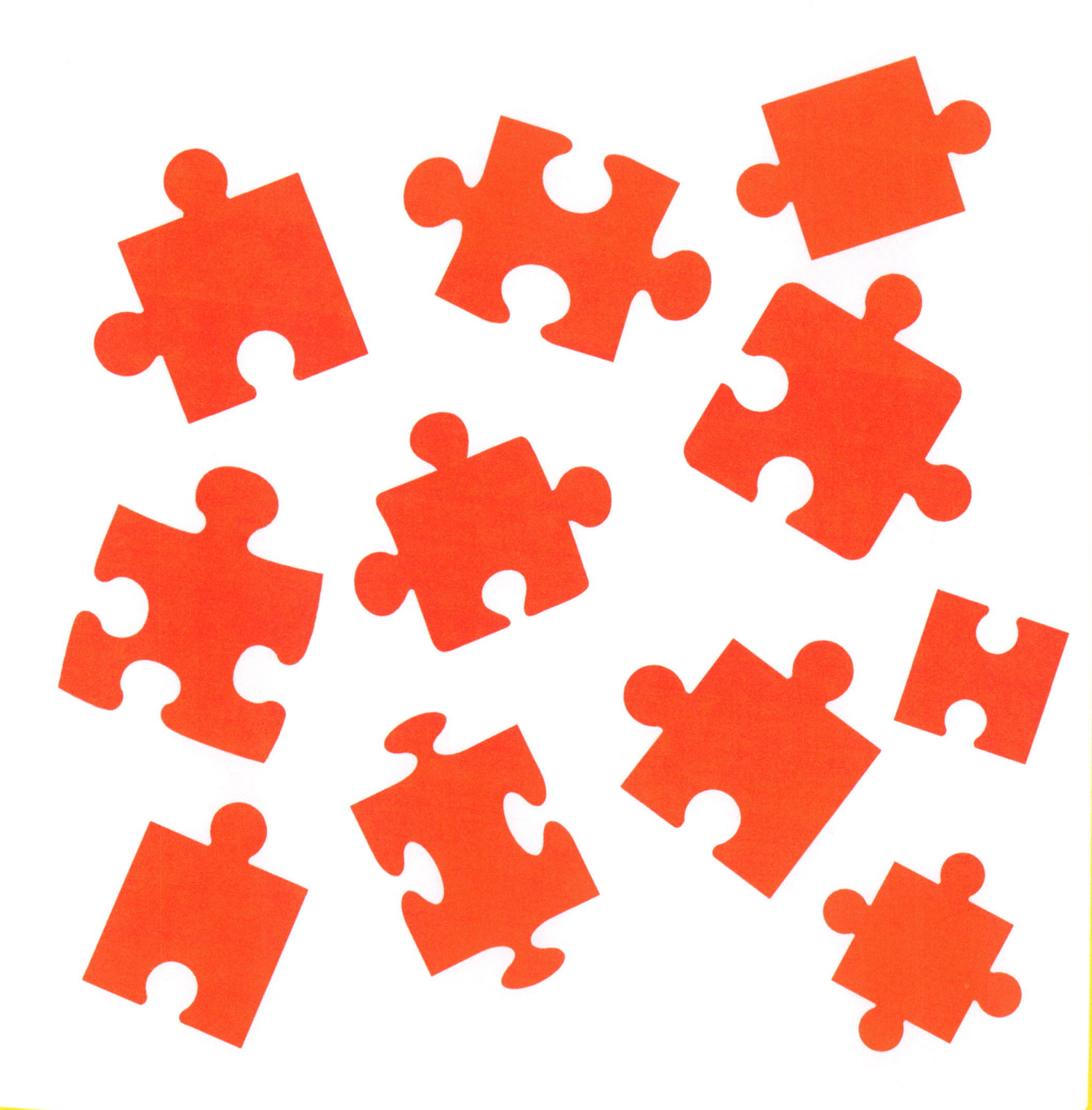

"Keep your mouth shut."

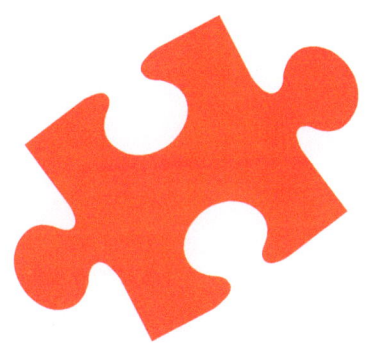
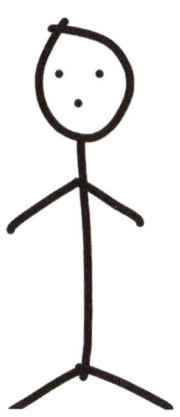

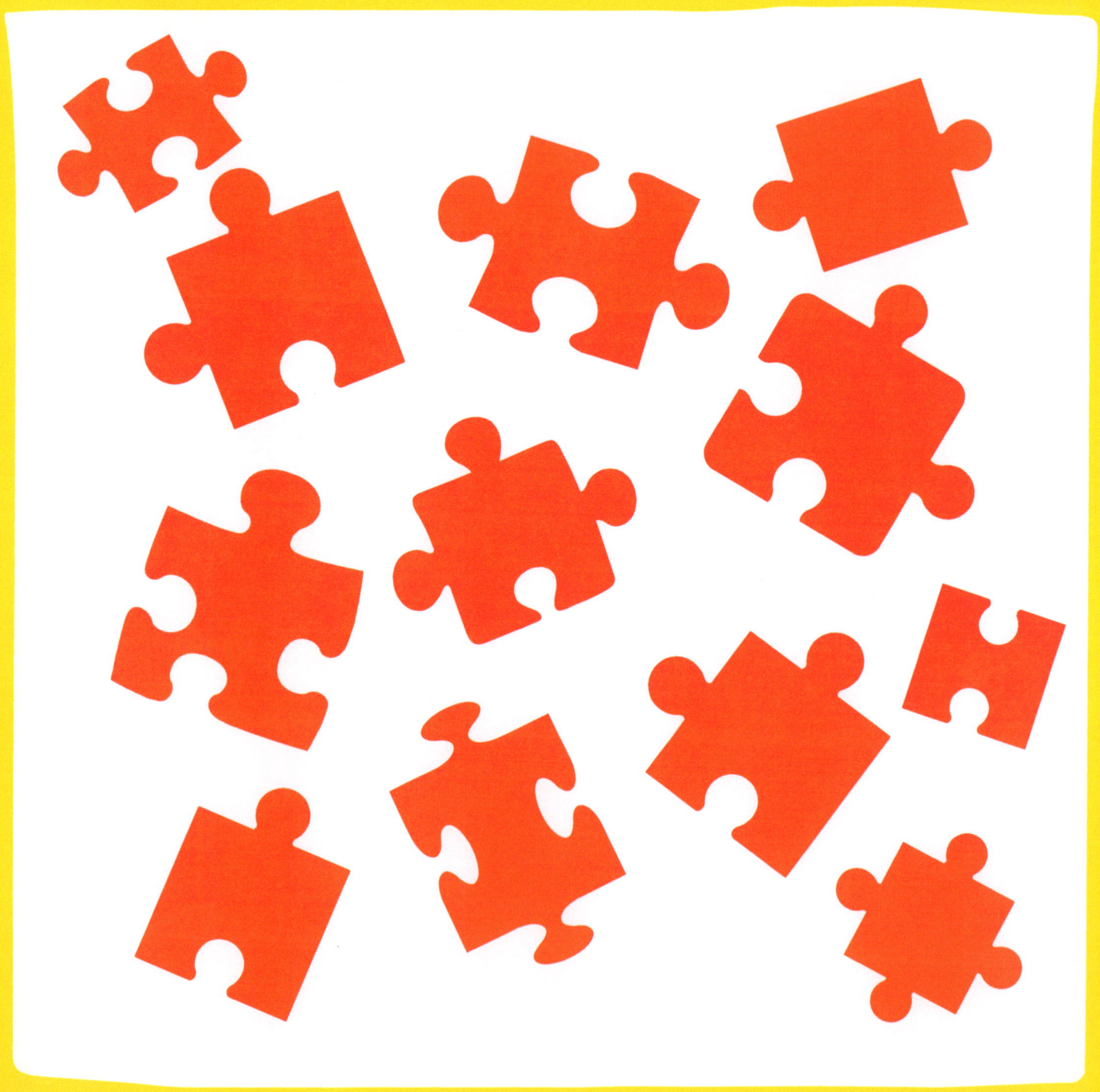

"I don't know why this is so hard for you."

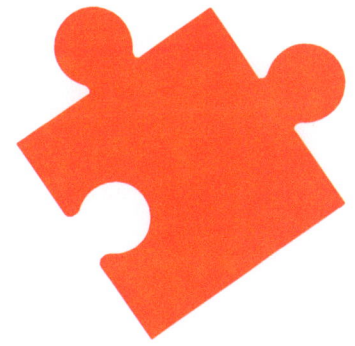

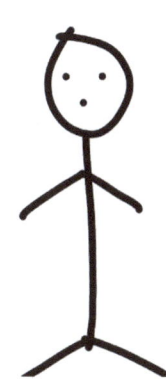

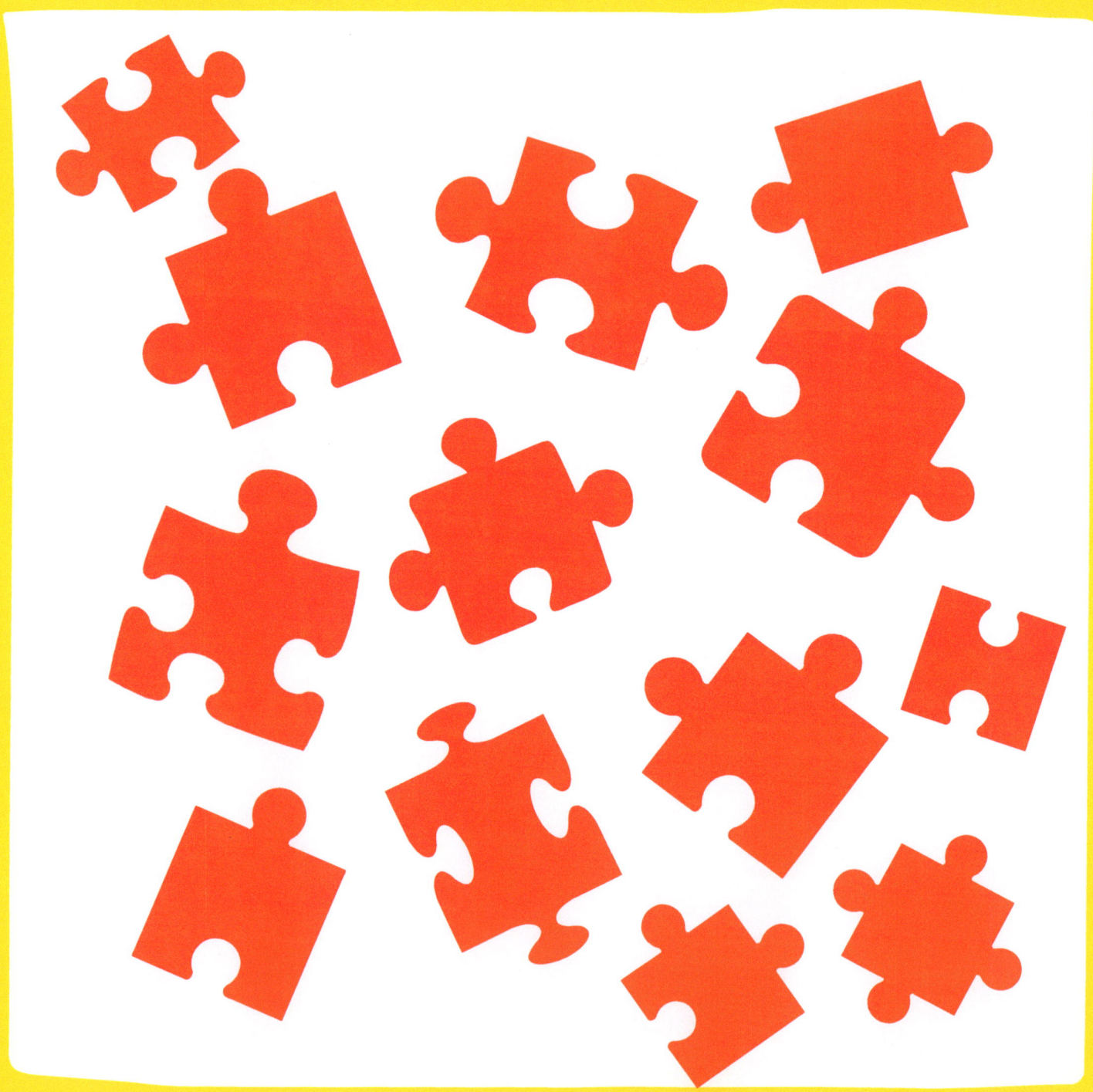

"You need help."

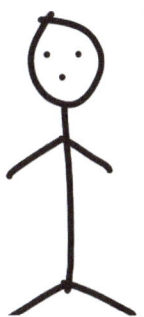

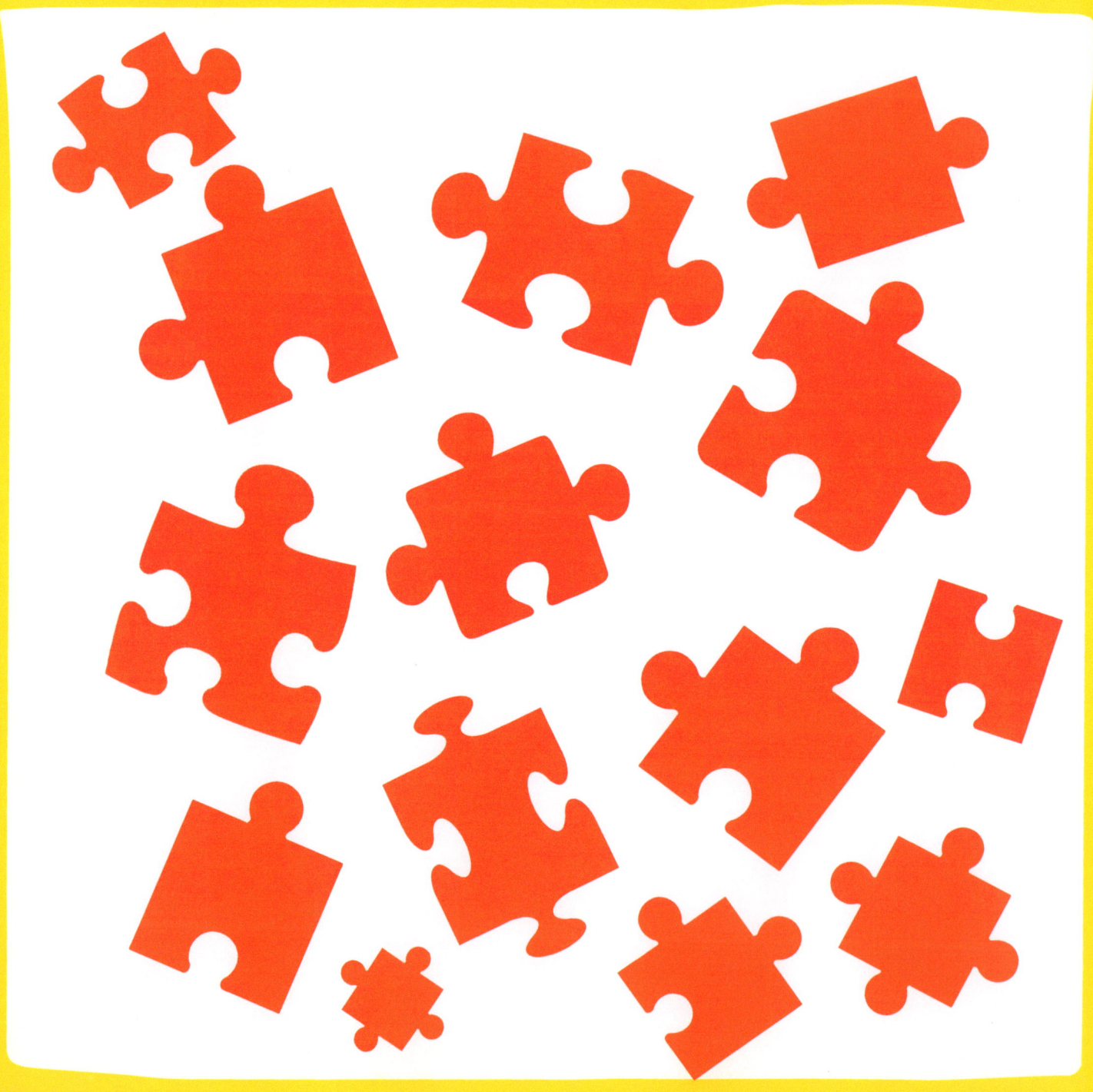

"Stop saying sorry."

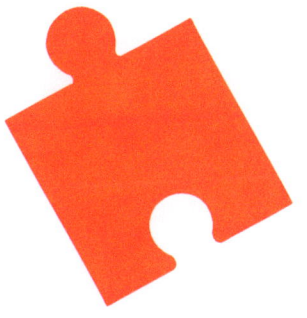
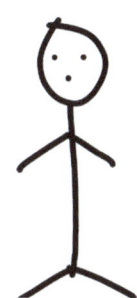

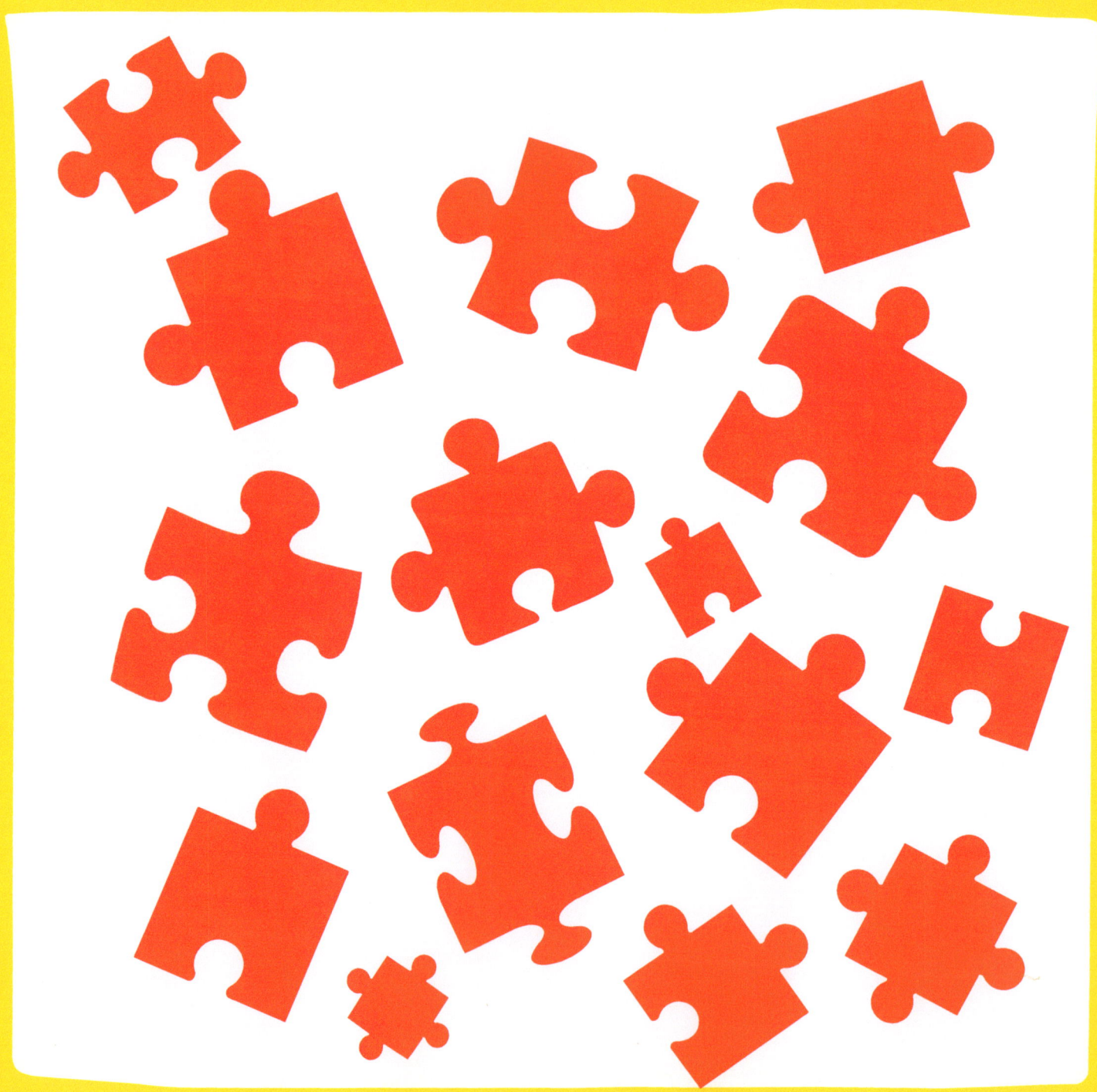

"You fail at everything."

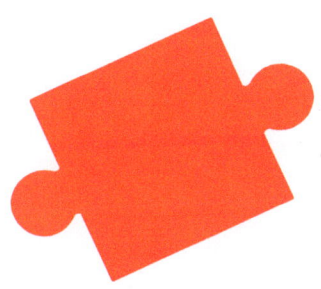

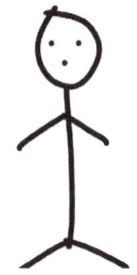

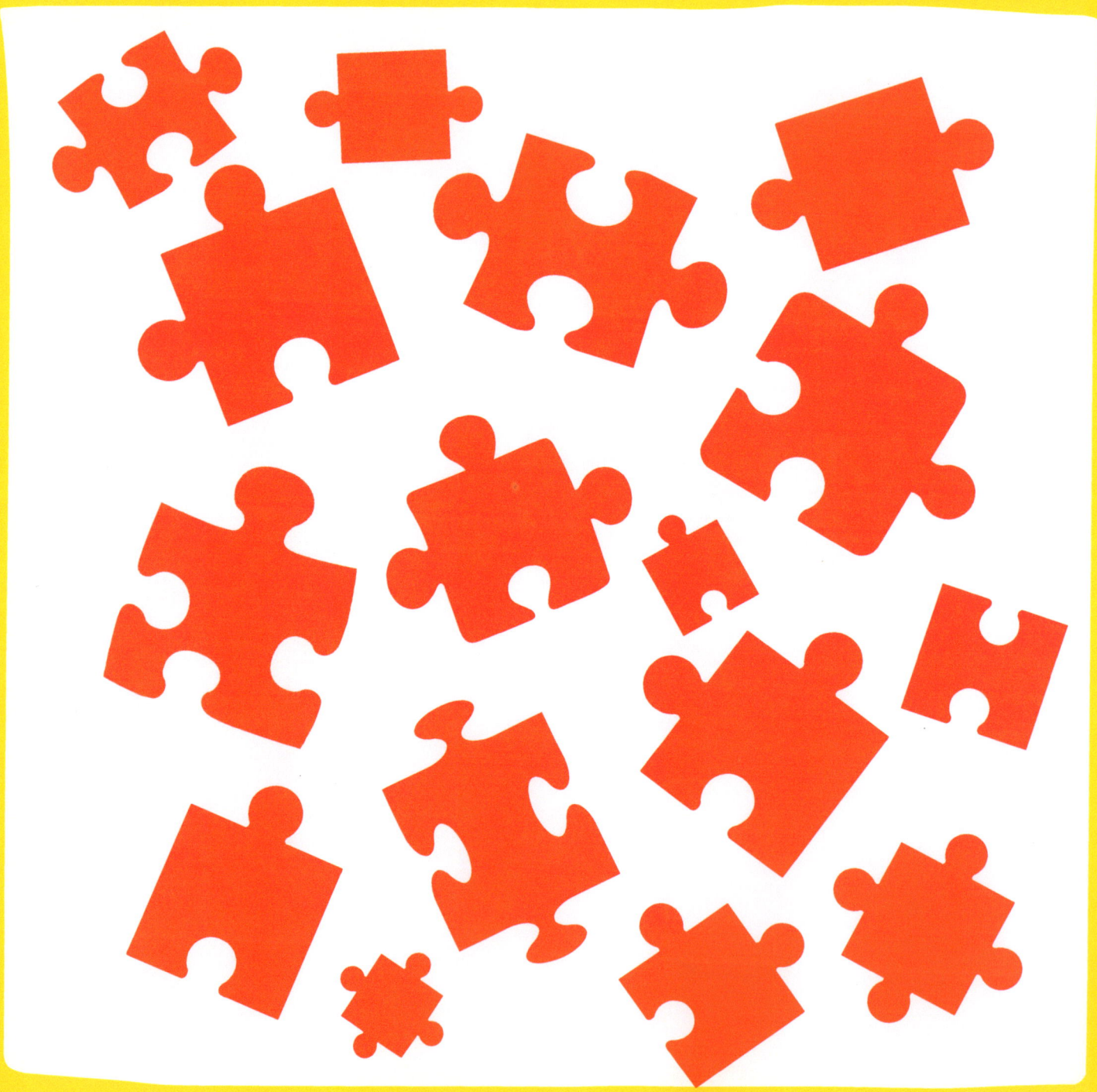

"How could you not know that?"

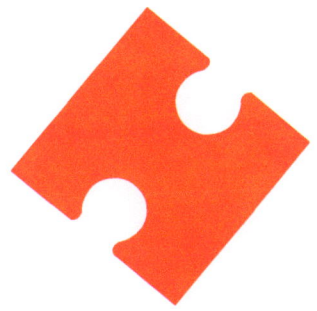

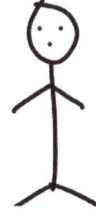

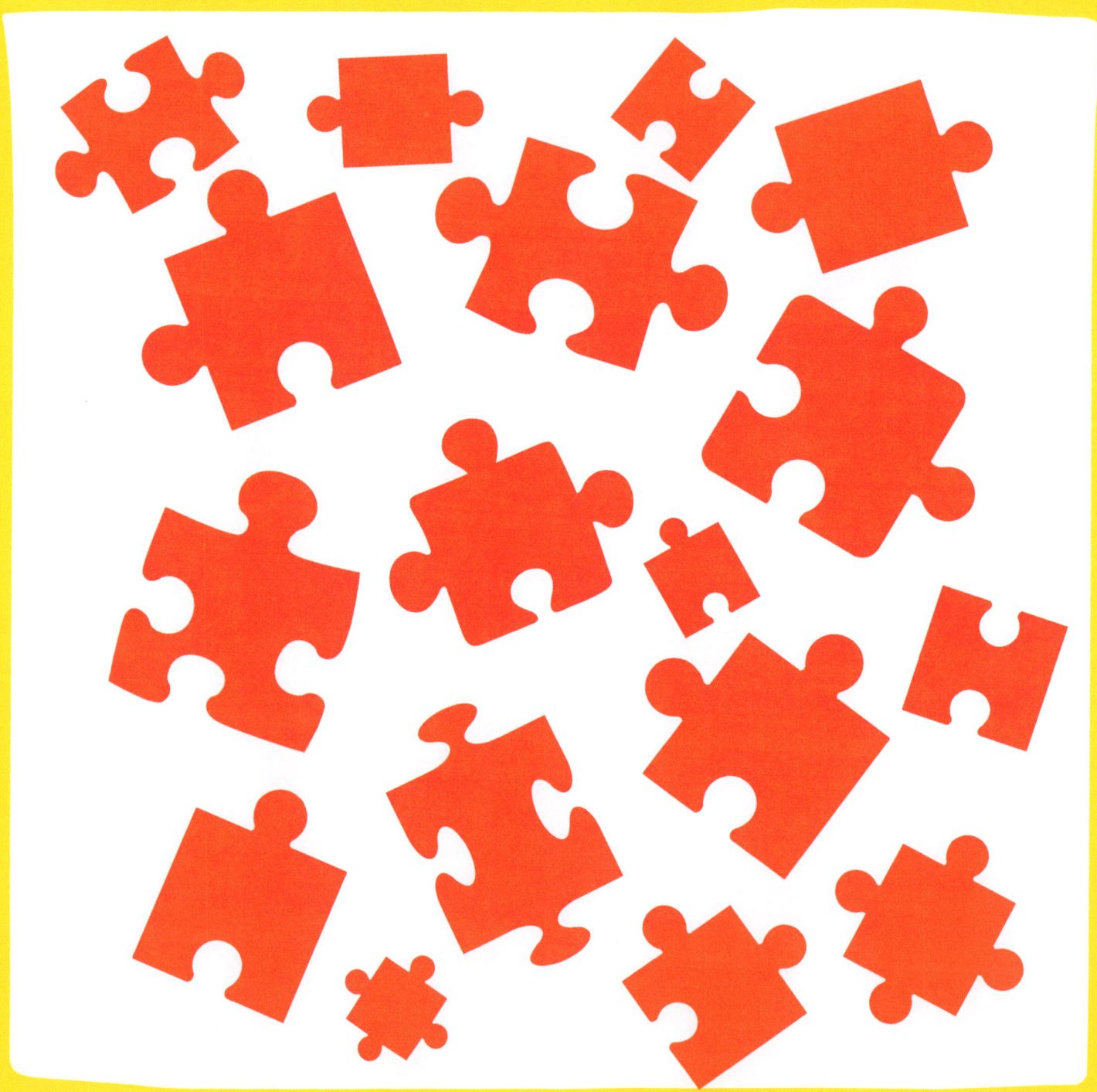

"You're embarrassing."

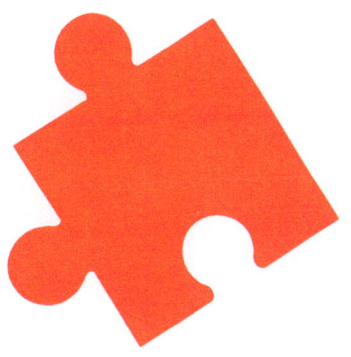

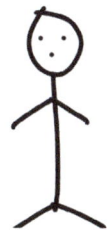

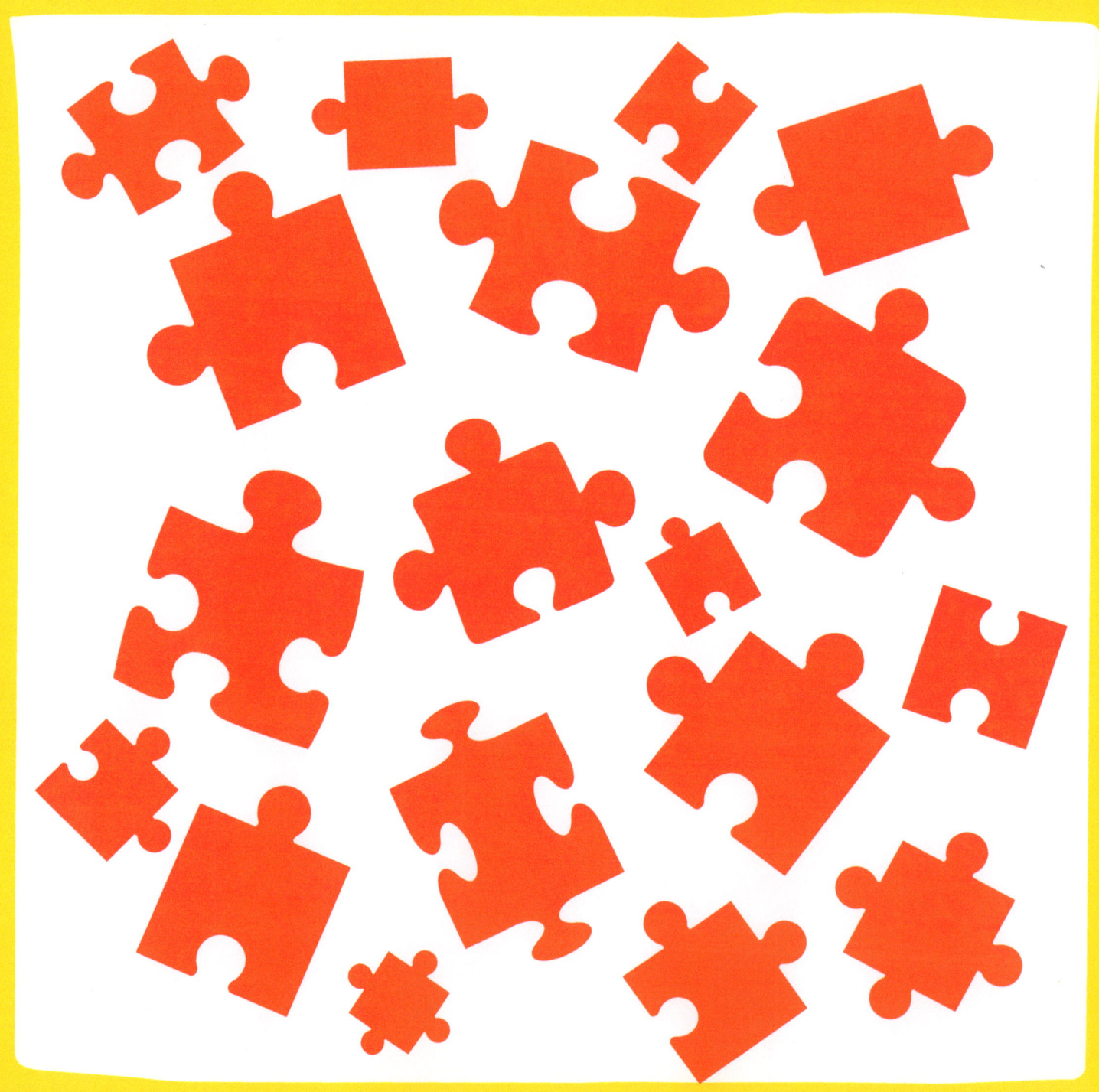

"I don't understand you."

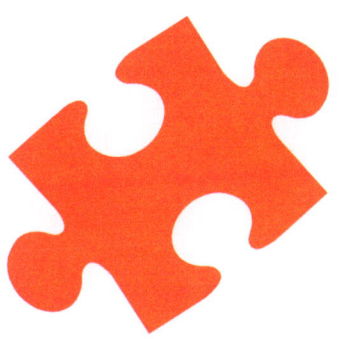

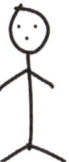

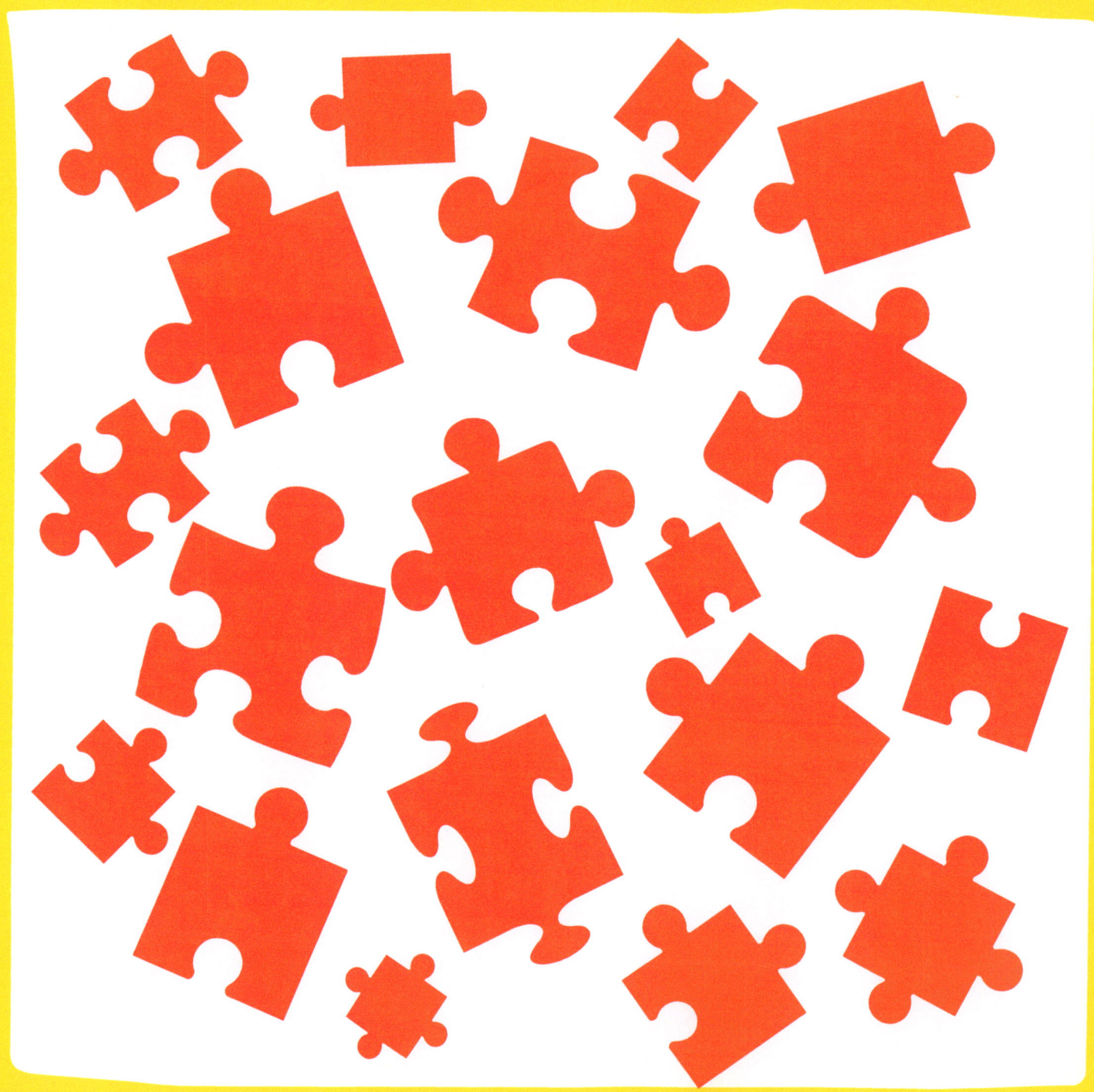

"You're too much."

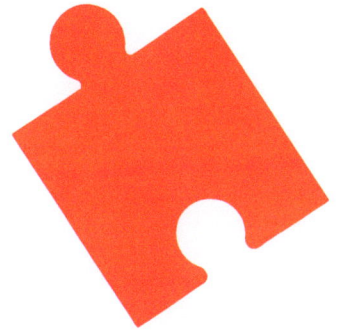

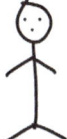

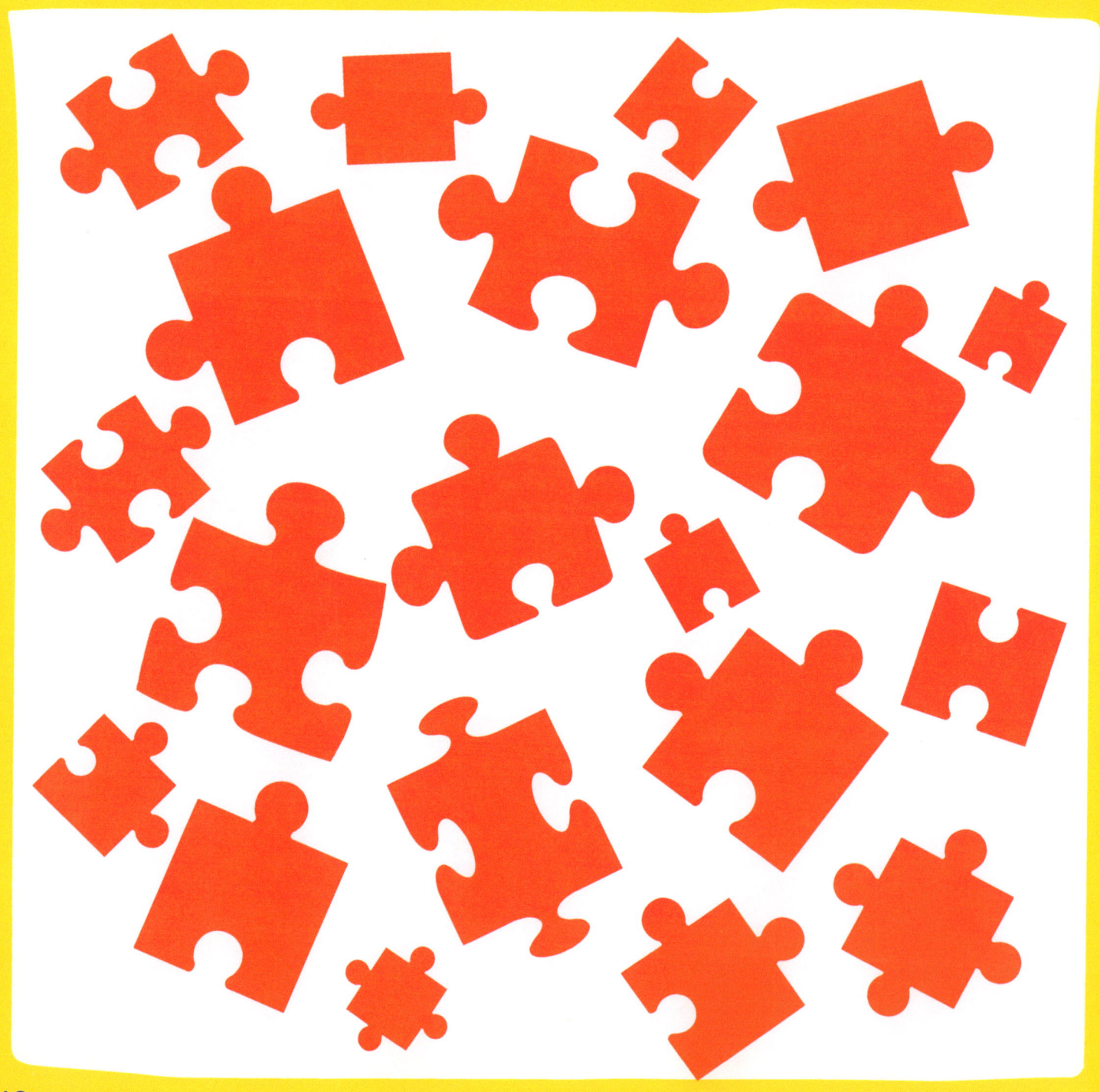

"You need to know your audience."

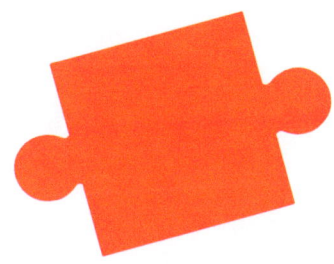

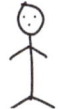

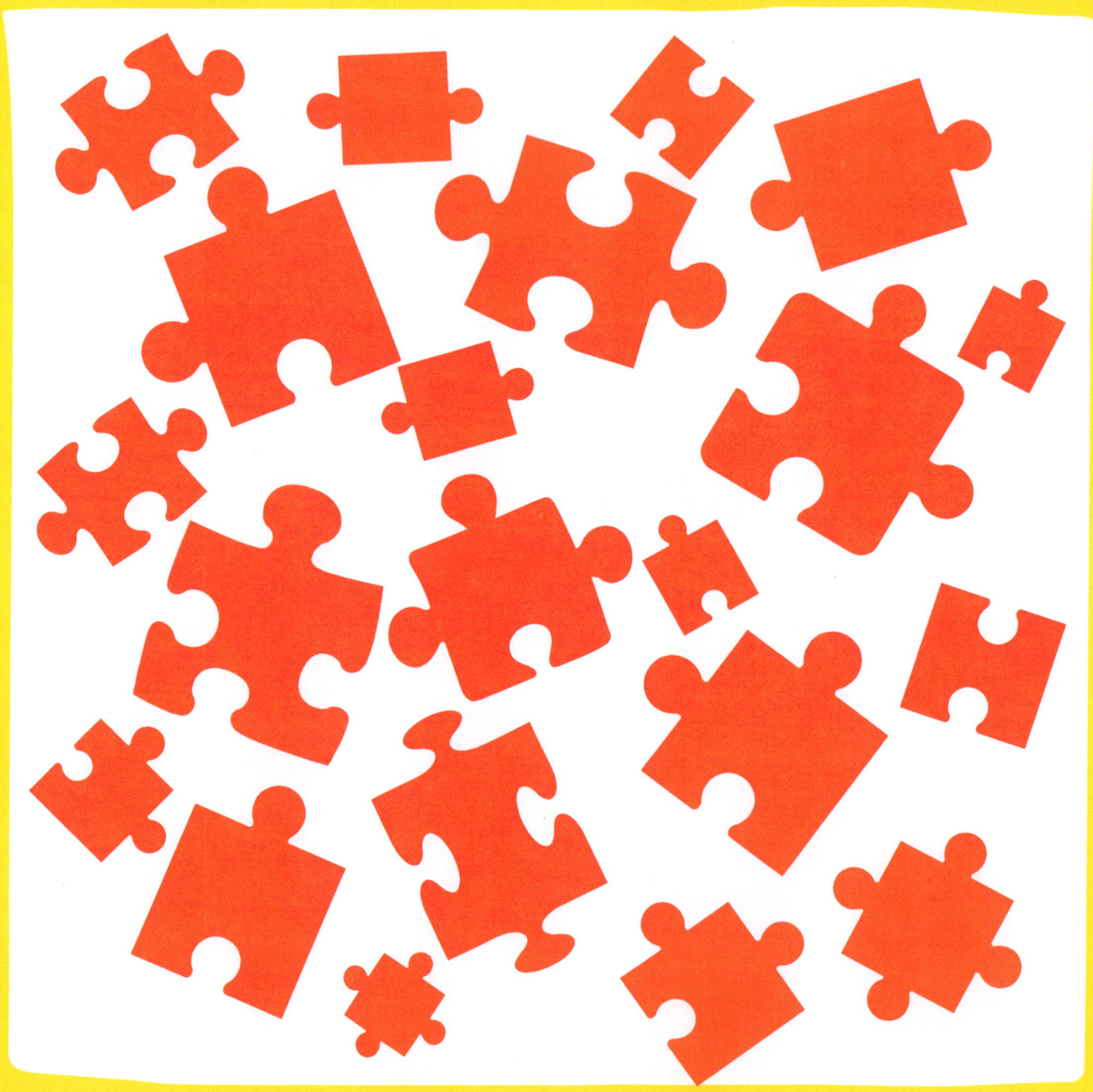

"You're a disappointment."

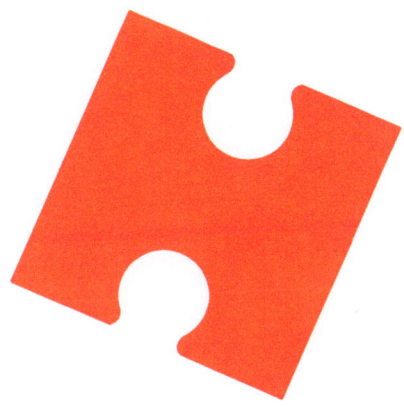

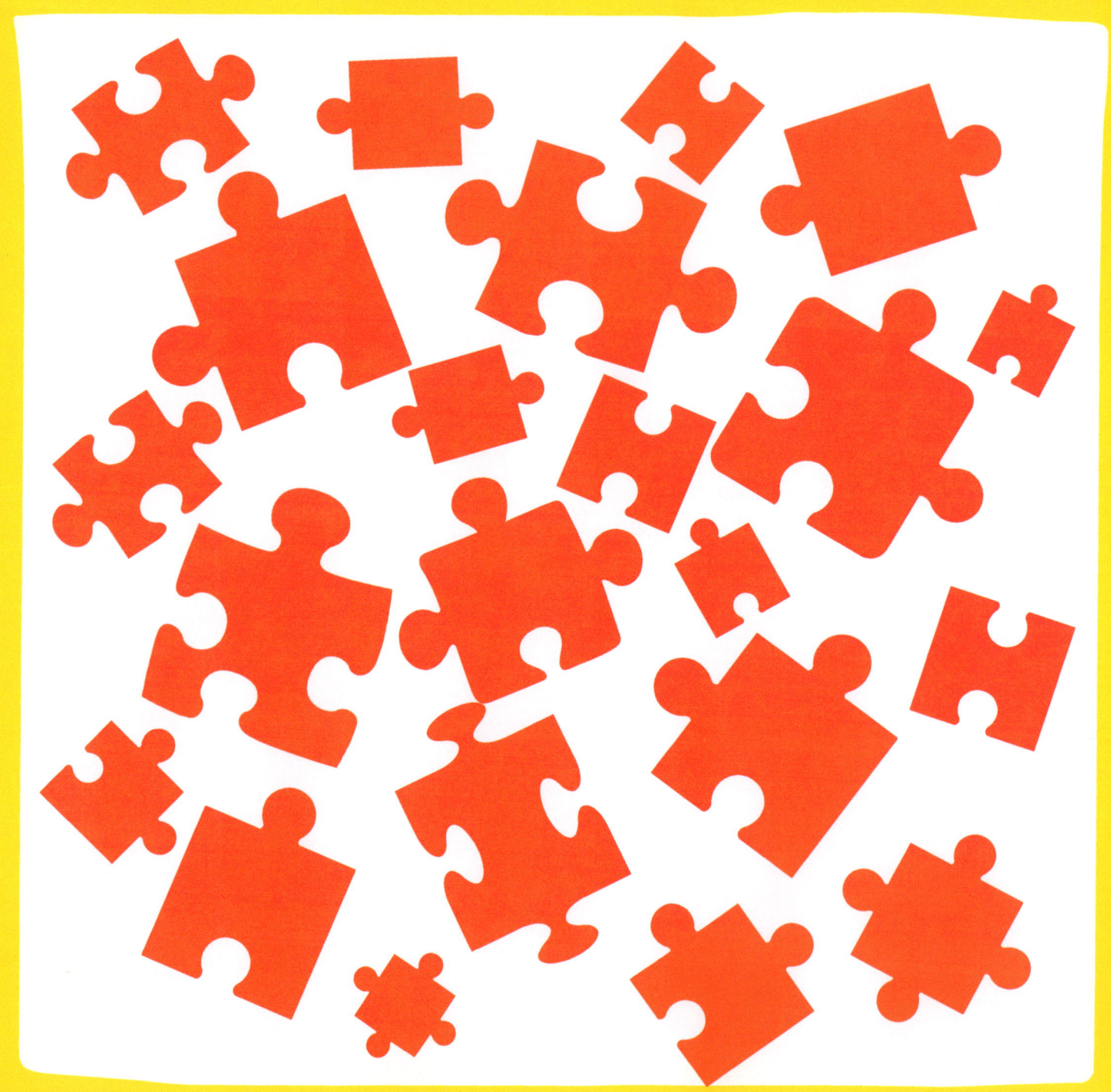

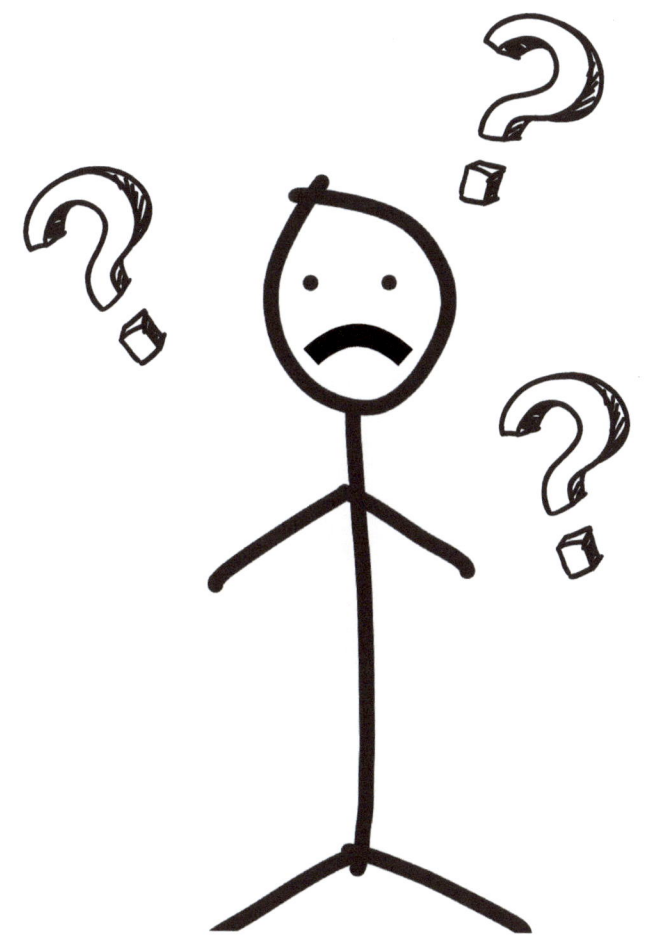

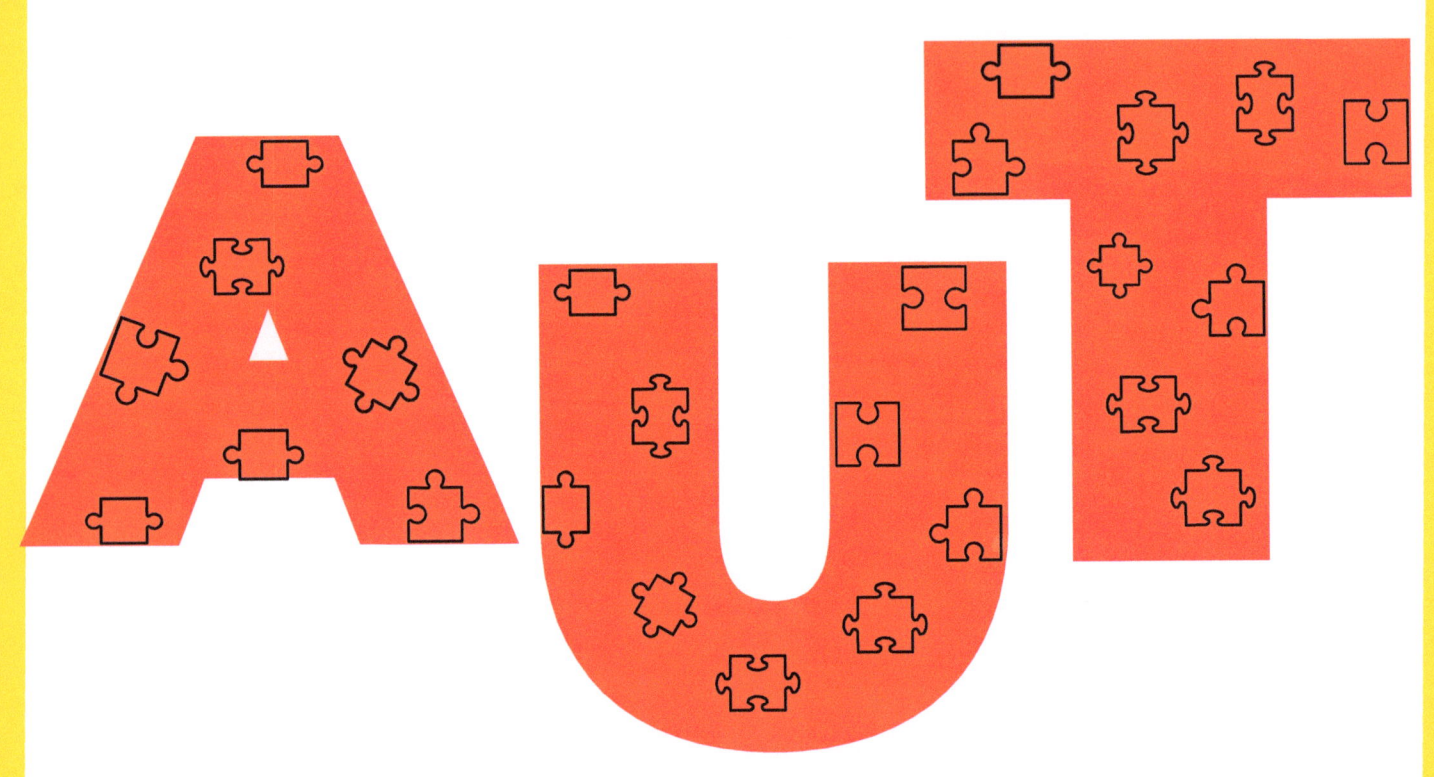

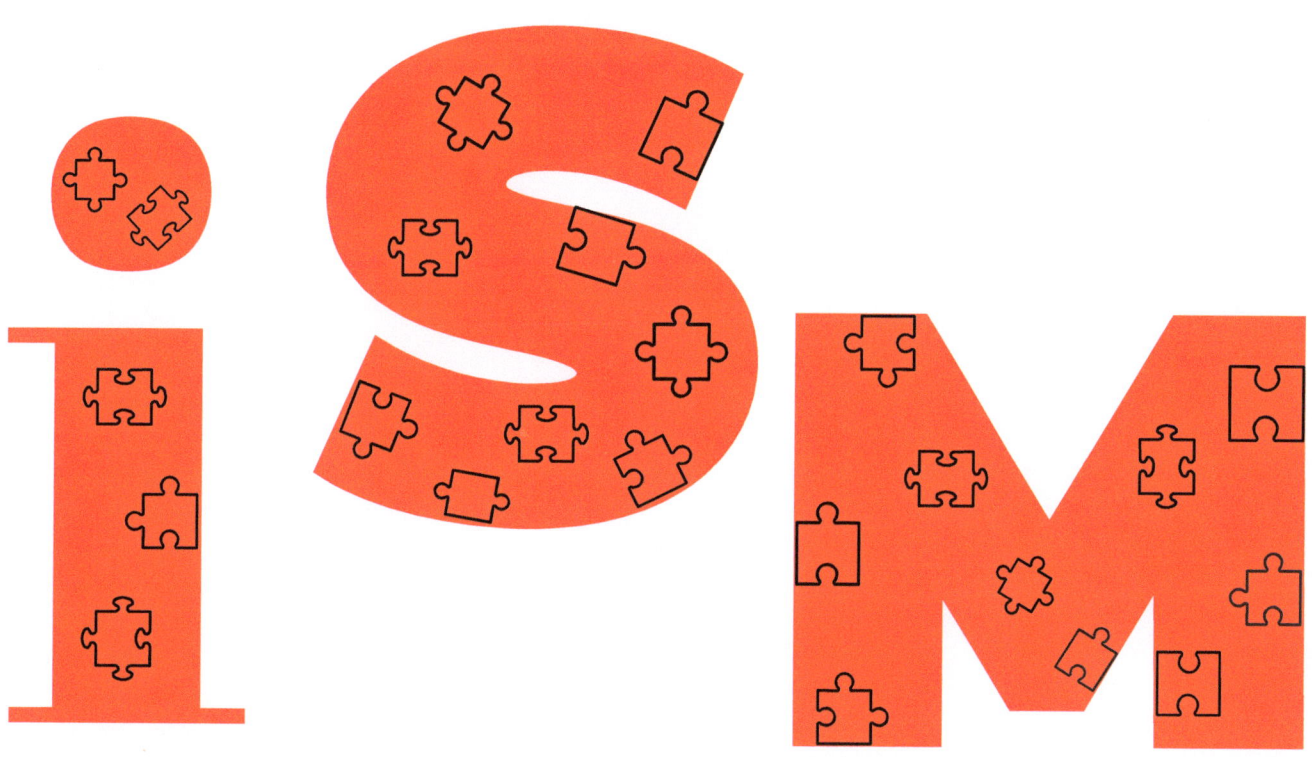

48

"Oh... Nothing."

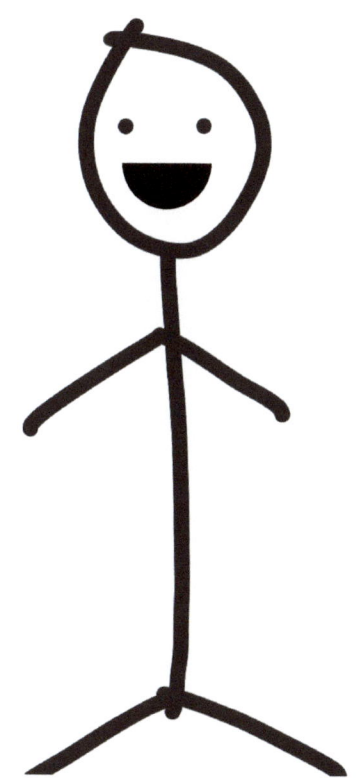

A Note From the Author

To some, this book might not seem like much. To me, it's the result of 35 years of extensive personal research and experience. I've heard every quote in this book thousands of times, in varying volumes, and with loads of profanity sprinkled in. I've collected these "moral failings" since childhood, hoping that one day I would finally have an answer to the question "what is wrong with me?"

Well, it turns out I'm autistic. And nothing is wrong with me.

Although autism means many things to many people, to me, my diagnosis means I no longer have to hate myself. That alone is a life-changing revelation. Instead of the ugly, deformed, weird, loud, embarrassing duck that I always thought I was, I am a beautiful, weird, smart, kind, bad-ass, autistic swan.

This revelation didn't fix my entire life, but it changed my future. I now wake up saying "what fun can I get into," or "I really hope I find a cool rock," instead of saying "let's try not to screw up too bad today."

By naming my "problem," I vanquished the shame, regret and self-hatred that has been a constant in my life. Instead, I actually like the person that I am for the very first time.

This book is my love letter to myself, and I only wish that I had written it sooner.

Autism Resources

According to the Centers for Disease Control and Prevention, autism affects and estimated 1 in 44 children and 1 in 45 adults in the United States today.

The following resources and organizations work tirelessly to help individuals affected by autism.

Autism Speaks
www.autismspeaks.org

Interactive Autism Network
www.iancommunity.org

Autism Society
www.autism-society.org

Autism Science Foundation
www.autismsciencefoundation.org

Interagency Autism Coordinating Committee
www.iacc.hhs.gov

Centers for Disease Control and Prevention
www.cdc.gov/ncbddd/autism/index.html

Nicole Yates

Nicole Yates lives with her husband, dog, and exorbitant number of cats In the middle of nowhere, Montana. She is an avid reader, fisherwoman, and cross-stitch extraordinaire. She writes about her life experience and hopes to share the lessons she has learned to help others.

"WHAT'S WRONG WITH YOU?"

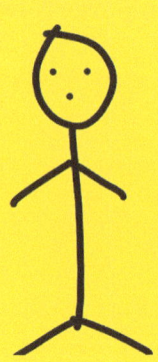

Approximately 2.2% of adults in the United States are on the autism spectrum.

Did you grow up feeling like you just couldn't fit in or that you didn't belong? Have you struggled to put together the pieces of why you couldn't just "be normal?"

What's Wrong With You is a simple story that navigates the experience of not fitting in and feeling small, until you are able to put all the pieces together to understand who you really are.

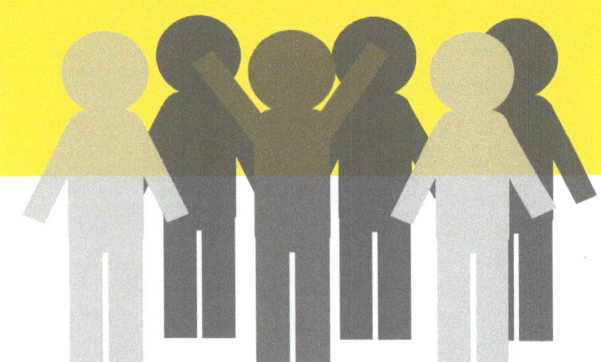

E. Rose Books

www.ingramcontent.com/pod-product-compliance
Lightning Source LLC
Chambersburg PA
CBHW051212220526
45473CB00003B/998